BRUSH, COMB, SCRUB
Inventions to Keep You Clean

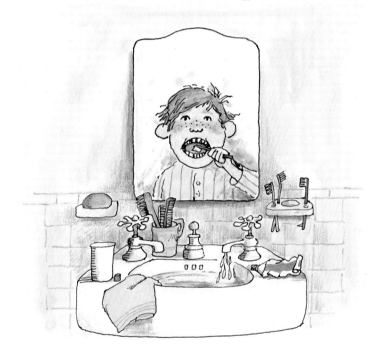

VICKI COBB
Pictures by Marylin Hafner

HarperTrophy
A Division of HarperCollins*Publishers*

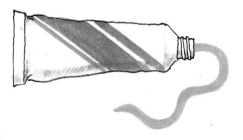

Library of Congress Cataloging-in-Publication Data
Cobb, Vicki.
    Brush, comb, scrub : inventions to keep you clean.

    Summary: Describes how soap and water, toothpaste and
toothbrush, and comb and brush were invented and how they
keep us clean and healthy.
    1. Hygiene products—Juvenile literature.   2. Hygiene—
Juvenile literature.   [1. Cleanliness.   2. Grooming]
I. Hafner, Marylin, ill.   II. Title.
RA778.5.C63   1989   646.7'1'028   88-2930
ISBN 0-397-32312-3
ISBN 0-397-32313-1 (lib. bdg.)
ISBN 0-06-446107-6 (pbk.)

First Harper Trophy edition, 1993.

KEEPING CLEAN

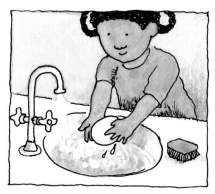

Wash your hands.

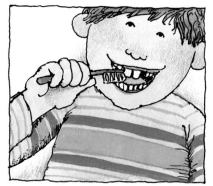

Brush your teeth.

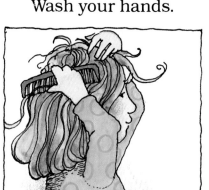

Comb your hair.

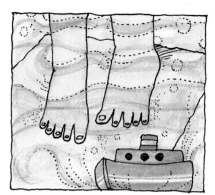

Take a bath.

Most people do these things at least once or twice a day.
But what if we didn't?

Dirt and sweat would collect on the skin. We would start to smell bad. We would get sores on our skin. Our hair would get matted and tangled. Our teeth would fall out. People who don't keep themselves clean get sick much more easily than people who do.

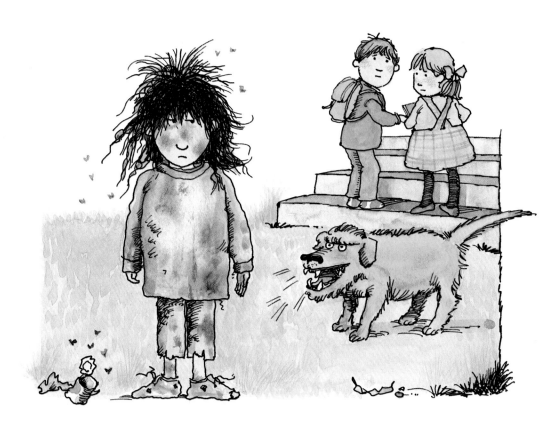

Today it's easy to clean yourself up.

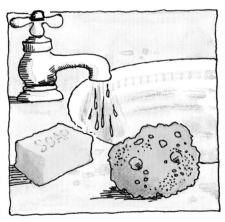

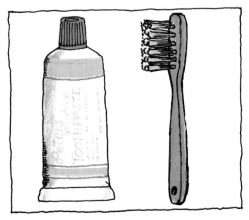

Soap and water,   toothpaste and toothbrush,

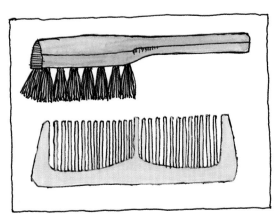

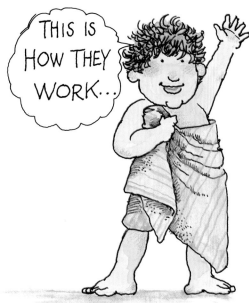

comb and brush, are all handy.

RUNNING WATER

Want to wash your hands? Go turn on the faucet. Out comes clean water. Dirty water disappears down the drain. Today about half the people in the world have hot and cold running water in their homes.

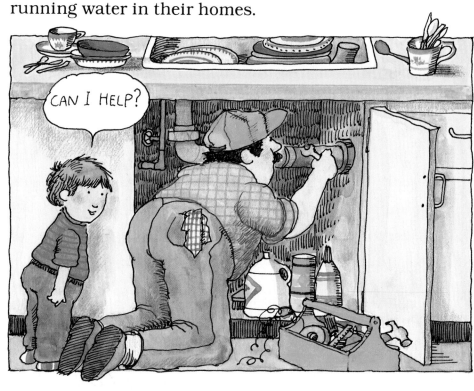

The pipes that bring clean water to your house and carry away waste water are called *plumbing*.

There are many places in the world where there is no plumbing. People have to carry in pails of water from a well or river or stream to take a bath. They have to heat the water on a fire.

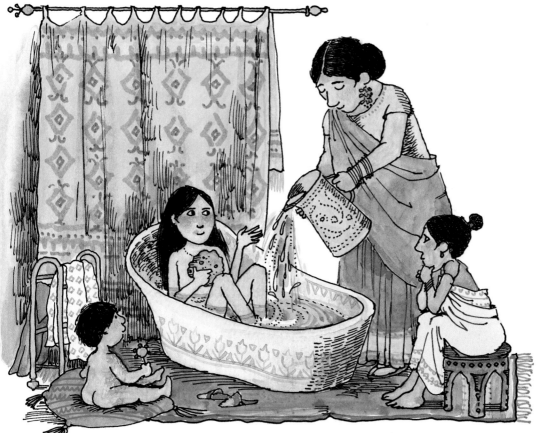

They may pour the water into a tub. A family may take turns using the same bathwater.

If you live in a city or town, your water may come from a river or lake. It goes through huge pipes to a special plant that makes it clean before it is piped to homes.

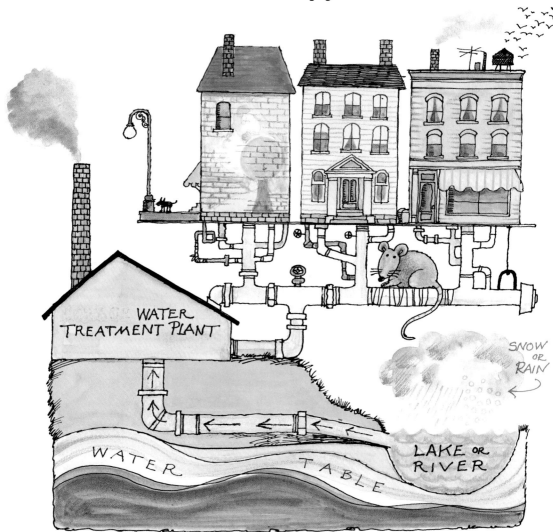

If you live in the country, your water probably comes from a well. A well is a deep hole in the ground that reaches pure, clean underground water.

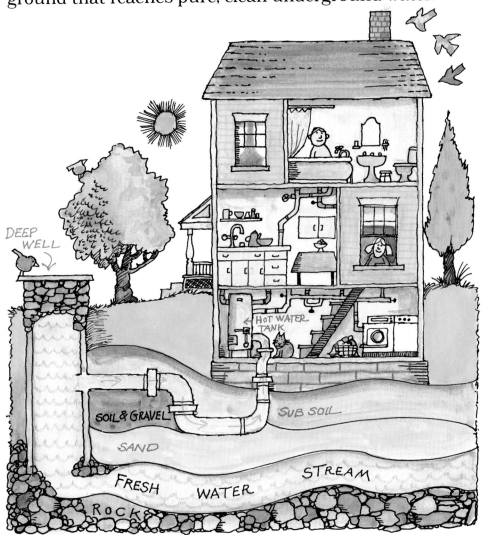

Here's how modern plumbing works. A pipe carrying clean water comes into your house from your water supply.

Some of the clean water goes into a heating tank called a *hot-water heater*. Both hot and cold water travel through pipes to sinks, showers, tubs, toilets, and washing machines.

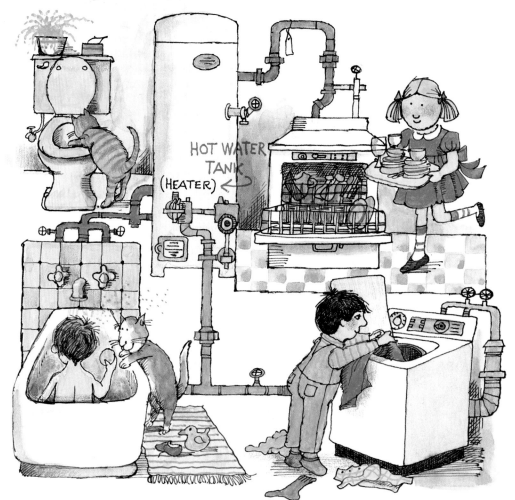

HOT WATER TANK (HEATER)

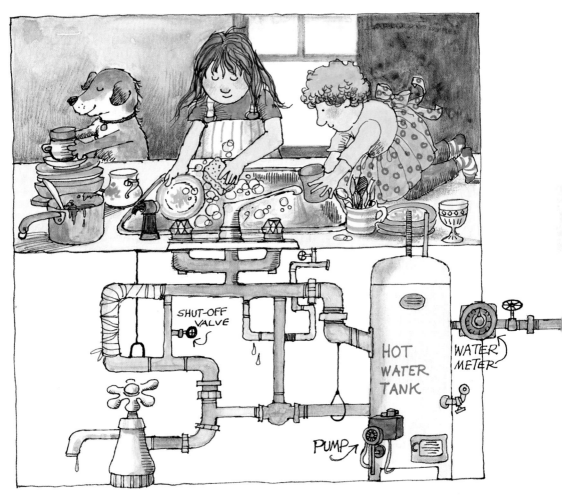

Machines called *pumps* push water through pipes. Clean water pushes against closed faucets. The push of the water is called water pressure. When you turn on a faucet, pumps make the water rush out.

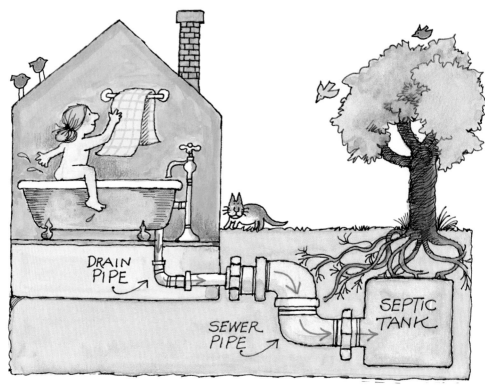

Waste water goes down into a different set of pipes, called *drainpipes*. All the drainpipes empty into one large drainpipe, which leaves your house and carries waste water into a sewer or septic tank.

Modern plumbing is set up so that clean water won't get mixed with waste water.

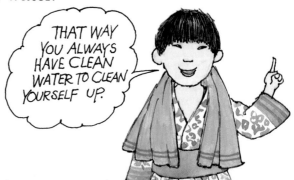

THAT WAY YOU ALWAYS HAVE CLEAN WATER TO CLEAN YOURSELF UP.

SOAP

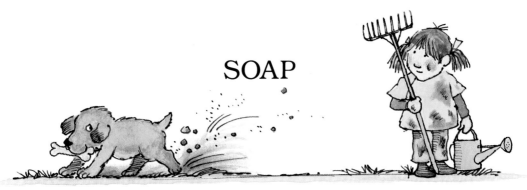

Water alone won't get you very clean. To wash yourself really well you need soap. Here's why. Skin has oil in it. Dirt often has grease in it. Water doesn't mix with oil or grease, but soap mixes with both. When you lather up your skin, the soap mixes with oil and grease. The dirt and oil are lifted from the skin. Then rinse water washes everything away.

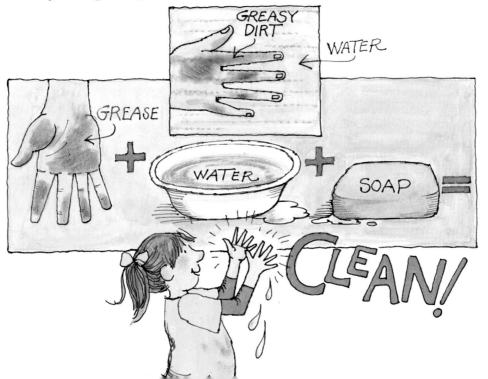

Soap was accidently discovered by the Romans about 3,000 years ago. Animal fat had dripped into the ashes of a fire. Rain washed the fat-and-ashes mixture into the river, where women were doing laundry. They pounded their laundry with rocks to get it clean. The women discovered that the mixture of ashes and fat and water helped get their clothes cleaner than pounding alone.

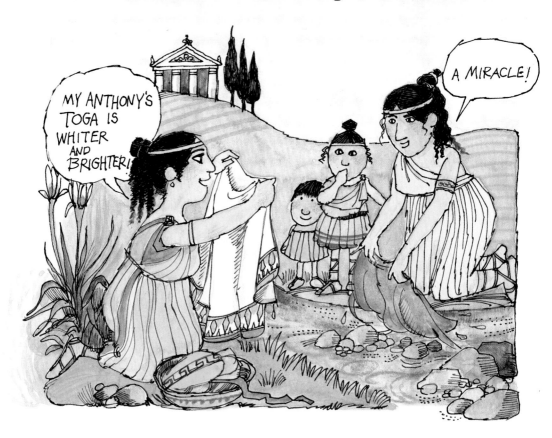

But no one used this early soap to clean the skin because it made the skin sore.

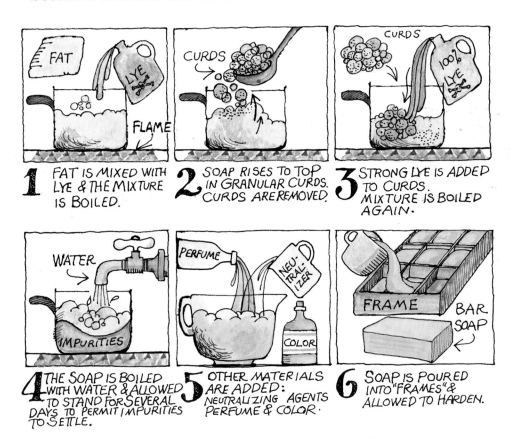

1 FAT IS MIXED WITH LYE & THE MIXTURE IS BOILED.

2 SOAP RISES TO TOP IN GRANULAR CURDS. CURDS ARE REMOVED.

3 STRONG LYE IS ADDED TO CURDS. MIXTURE IS BOILED AGAIN.

4 THE SOAP IS BOILED WITH WATER & ALLOWED TO STAND FOR SEVERAL DAYS TO PERMIT IMPURITIES TO SETTLE.

5 OTHER MATERIALS ARE ADDED: NEUTRALIZING AGENTS PERFUME & COLOR.

6 SOAP IS POURED INTO "FRAMES" & ALLOWED TO HARDEN.

Later people learned to make soap by cooking oils or fats in a very strong, poisonous chemical called *lye*. A kind of lye is found in ashes. Soap making is dangerous, messy, and smelly.

For hundreds of years people made soap at home. Home-made soap was strong. It was not pleasant to bathe with.

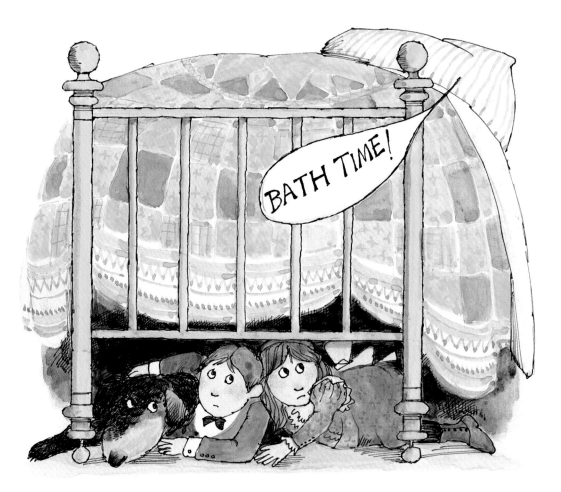

Then soap making became a business. Soap companies made it cheaper and easier to buy soap.

They made sweet-smelling, gentle soap for bathing. They made shampoos, liquid soap, soap flakes, and strong detergents for laundry. Today there's a different soap for every kind of washing job you can imagine.

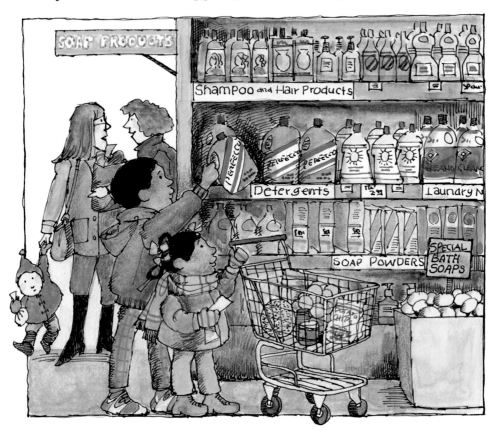

So when it's time to clean up, be sure to have some soap handy.

COMB AND BRUSH

Imagine how you would look if you never washed or combed or brushed your hair. A bird's nest would be neater! If you left your hair alone for only a few days, it would get knotted and matted. Try and comb it.

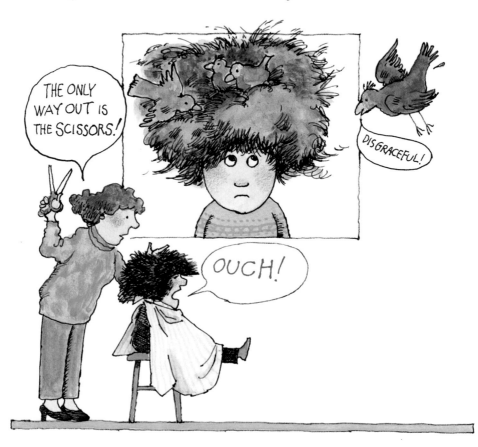

A brush will get out snarls and knots. It has dozens of stiff bristles that are pushed through your hair. Brushing removes hair that is about to fall out. You shed about one hundred hairs a day. But don't worry. About one hundred new hairs start growing every day to take their place.

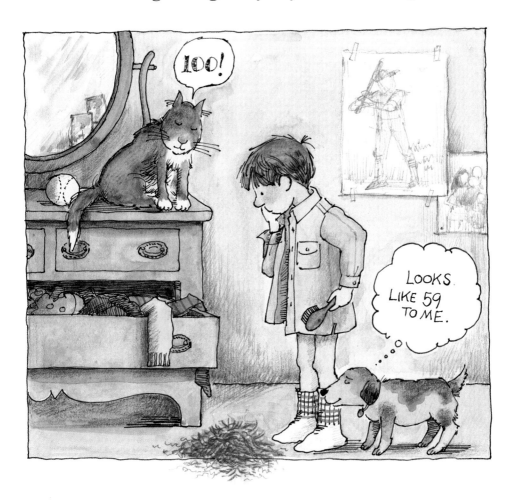

Brushing makes your hair silky, because it spreads oil from your scalp through your hair. It also makes your scalp tingle. Some people with long hair may brush fifty strokes or more a day to keep their hair beautiful.

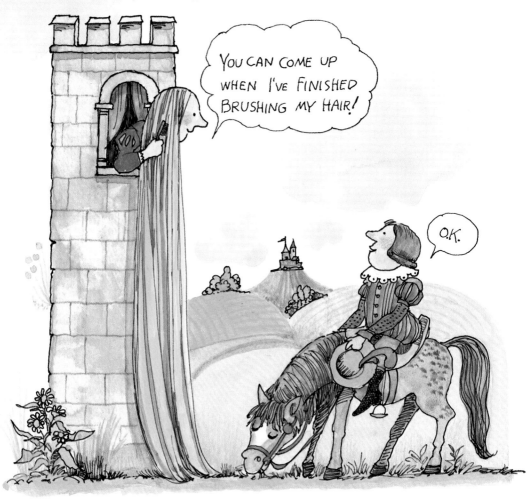

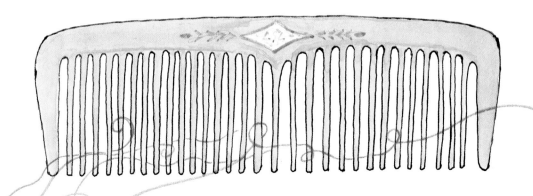

No one knows who invented the comb. A comb is like a rake. The parts of a comb that rake your hair are called *teeth*. The teeth line up your hair in straight rows. They pull out small knots. But a brush works better for getting out knots than a comb because it has many more bristles than a comb has teeth.

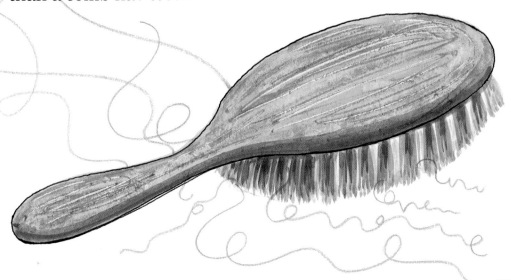

You use a comb to make your hair neat and to give it style. You can use a comb to divide your hair into parts.

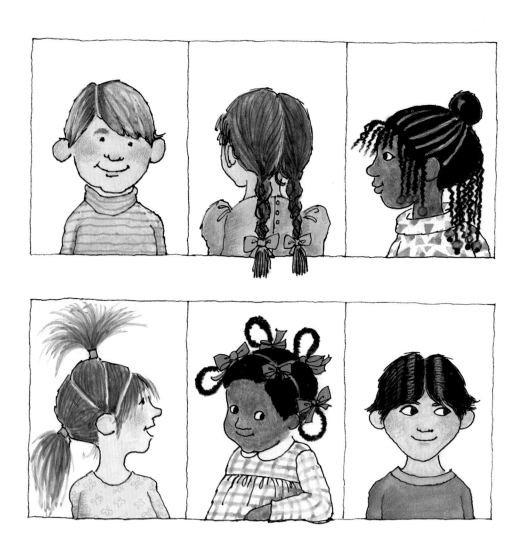

The first combs were fish bones or carved from wood.
Later people made them from shells and from ivory.

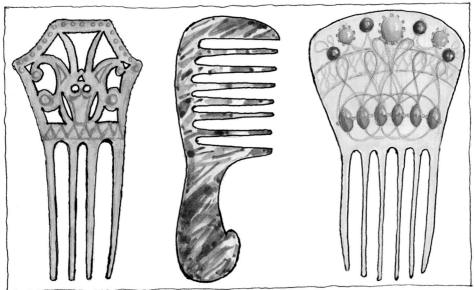

Today combs are made from hard rubber and from plastic.

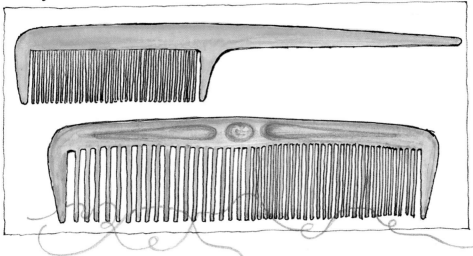

TOOTHBRUSH AND TOOTHPASTE

You know what happens if you don't brush your teeth daily. You get cavities and toothaches! Long ago, before there were toothbrushes and toothpaste, people probably only used toothpicks.

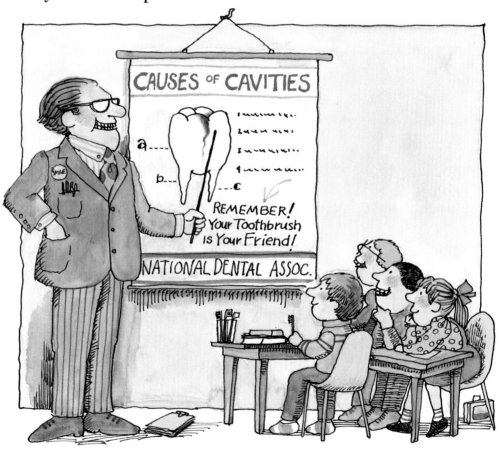

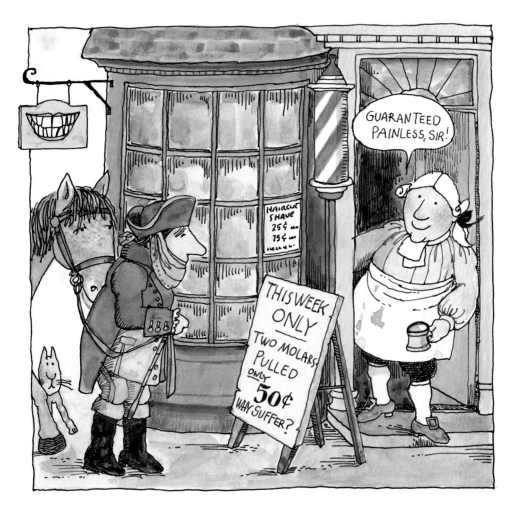

Sooner or later their teeth would rot. They got rid of toothaches by having teeth pulled. People expected to be toothless if they lived to old age. This still happens today to people who don't look after their teeth.

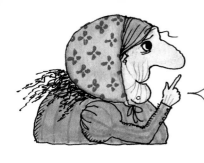

OVER THE YEARS PEOPLE CLEANED THEIR TEETH WITH:

ground-up chalk or charcoal,

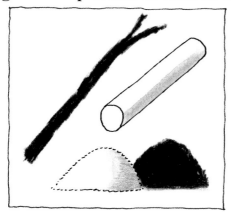

lemon juice,

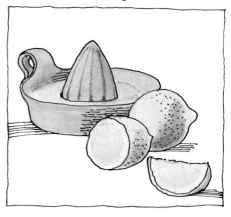

ashes,

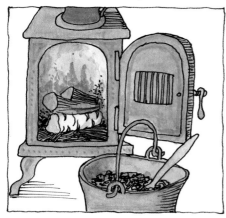

a mixture of tobacco and honey.

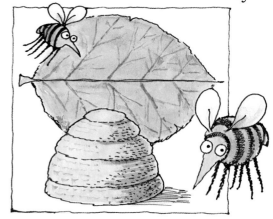

The first cream for cleaning teeth was made a little more than one hundred years ago. It was sold in jars. It did a good job when it was brushed on teeth. And best of all, it tasted minty.

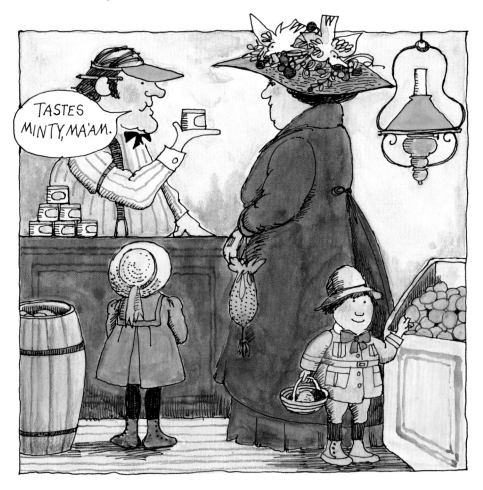

Then a toothpaste maker invented a tube that let you squeeze the toothpaste right onto the brush. The toothpaste tube was a great hit. More people began brushing their teeth.

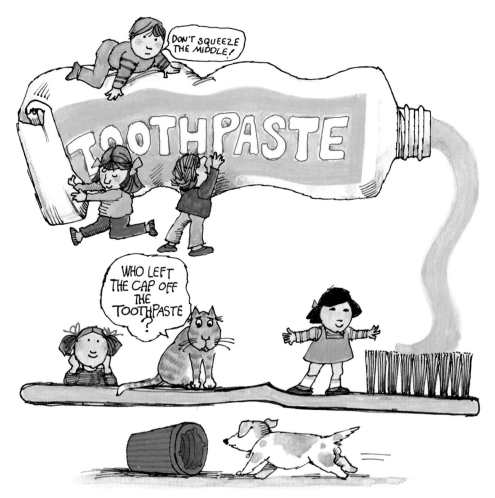

But brushing only became a habit in this country after World War II. The army gave toothbrushes and toothpaste to all its soldiers. The soldiers learned to brush twice a day.

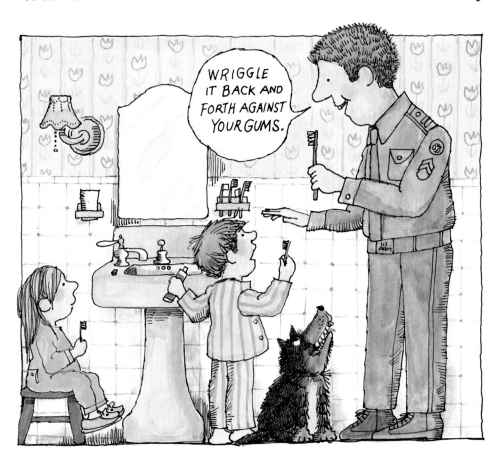

When the war was over, the soldiers went home and taught their families that brushing was important.

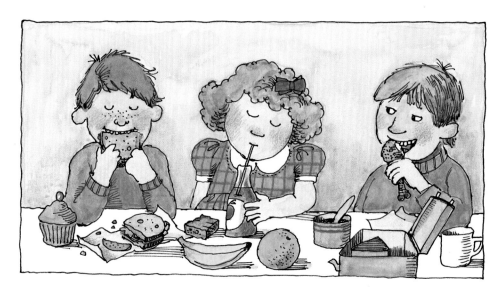

Here's the reason. Bits of food get caught in your teeth. There are germs on the food and in your mouth. If you don't keep brushing away the germs, they will grow in your mouth. The growing germs make liquids that can eat away the hard outer surface of your teeth. That's how you get cavities.

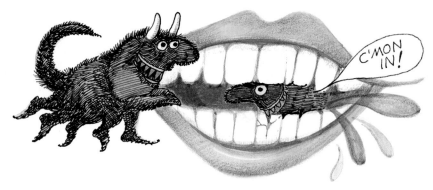

Brushing removes the food in your mouth that germs need to grow. It removes many of the germs. But you have to keep brushing regularly, because new germs enter your mouth with every meal.

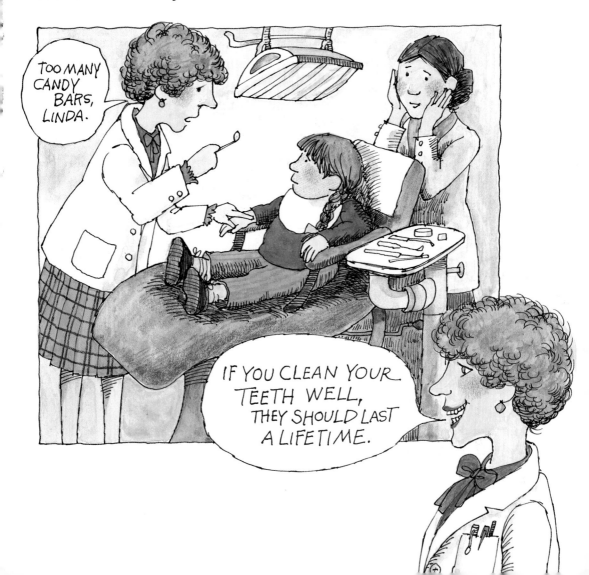

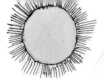

If you keep yourself clean, you will look good and feel good.

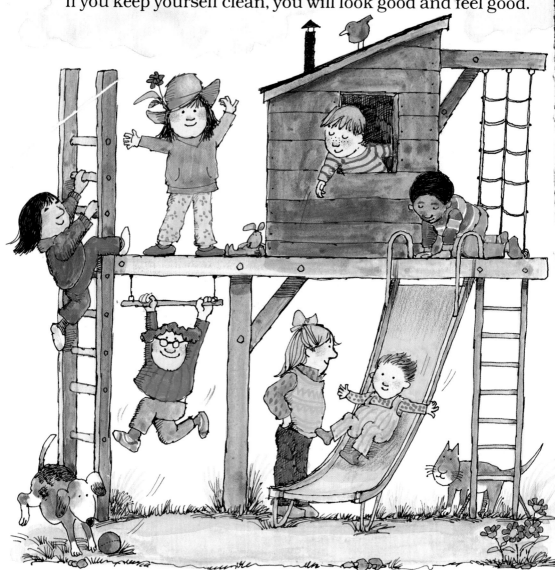

It's the healthful way to live.